ASTHMA WHO CARES?
- IN THE HOME

A manual to help parents
whose children have asthma

In children, asthma is twice as common in boys as in girls, so children with asthma are 'he' and 'him'.

ISBN 0 9520875 1 0

Reprinted February, 1993.

Reprinted & Revised August 1995.

INTRODUCTION

Many of you who have children with asthma are very aware of the need to learn more about the condition. It is for you that this book has been written.

We have endeavoured to cover most aspects of childhood asthma including the diagnosis and the various triggers that might cause your child's symptoms. We have looked at all the modern asthma treatments available, and the importance of preventive care, as well as all the different inhaler devices. We have spent time looking at how you, the parent can help your child manage his or her own asthma, by recording peak flow measurements and adjusting treatment when and where necessary.

Guidelines have been given on what to do if your child has an asthma attack, and on how to approach the school teacher in order to discuss your child's asthma management during school hours.

Above all I hope we have shown you that with guidance from your doctor and asthma nurse you can be largely responsible for providing the good care that your child deserves. If you can achieve this, you should be able to ensure that your child lives a happy, active, symptom free life for the great majority of the time.

Greta Barnes
Director
National Asthma Training Centre
August 1995

CONTENTS

YOUR CHILD AND ASTHMA

Could it be Asthma?

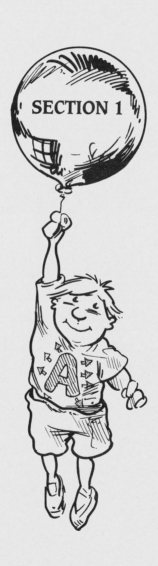

SECTION 1

1: COULD IT BE ASTHMA?

Asthma is very common, but these days it can be treated very effectively. Unfortunately many children get inadequate treatment for their asthma, or no treatment at all, because the diagnosis of asthma is not made.

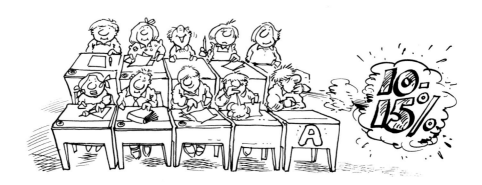

COMMON ... AND GETTING MORE COMMON

Lots of children have asthma. It is an accepted medical fact that in any large sample of school-aged children, 10-15% will have suffered asthma symptoms in the last year. There is also evidence that asthma is becoming more common, and more severe, although nobody is certain why. Research is going on into the links between asthma trends and environmental pollution, but so far no hard information is available.

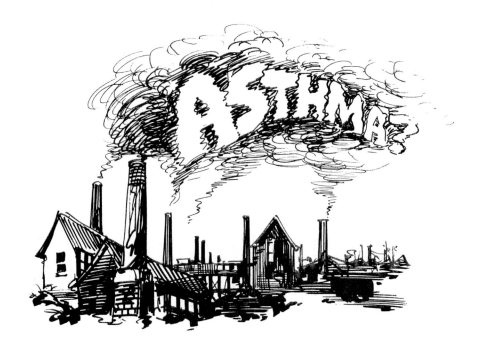

Although it may seem 'common sense' to think that air pollution and asthma must be linked, it might not be so simple. New Zealand is not noted for industrial pollution, but has more asthma sufferers per head of population than any other developed country.

> **A Definition:**
> "Asthma is an inflammation of the airways which is common and persistent. This inflammation causes variable obstruction and irritability of the airways, leading to cough, wheeze and tightness of the chest, often worse at night".

YOUR DOCTOR MAY NOT KNOW

As many as half of all children with asthma may not have been diagnosed as having asthma by their GP, so if your child has asthma, there's a good chance that you will be the one who spots it, not your family doctor. This doesn't mean your GP is incompetent - it's just that diagnosing asthma properly takes up a lot of time, more than the usual 5 to 10 minute appointment, and time is something that hard pressed GPs don't have. The doctor can't be blamed if patients just put up with their symptoms and don't go to the doctor.

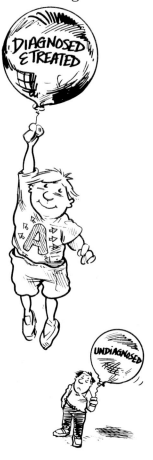

Strange as it may seem, you as a parent, even without medical training, may be able to spot asthma in your child more easily than your doctor, simply because you spend more time with him. You see him when he's ill, but the doctor only sees him in the surgery by which time, as often happens with asthma, he's fully recovered. Of course if you suspect asthma, you should tell your GP and ask him to investigate.

Being diagnosed as asthmatic by your doctor is important - without it your child won't get the right treatment.

SYMPTOMS TO LOOK OUT FOR

The main symptoms are **cough, wheeze and shortness of breath**. Wheeze is easy to recognise, and everybody associates it with asthma. Being short of breath is also pretty obvious, and well-recognised as an asthma symptom in children. Cough is a lot trickier, because sometimes it's the only symptom of asthma in children, and most parents, as well as many GPs, automatically think 'cough, therefore chest infection'. In fact asthma is the commonest cause of recurrent childhood cough.

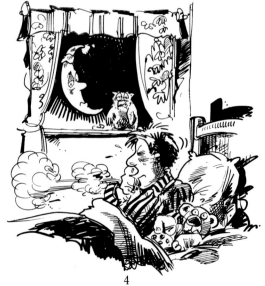

SLEEP

Asthma symptoms are variable and tend to be worse at night or in the early hours of the morning. If a child (or you!) is woken by coughing at night, asthma is one of the most likely causes.

EXERCISE

When children with asthma run around, they may cough or wheeze and get more breathless more quickly than other children. They also become more breathless, after they have stopped running around: this is typical of asthma.

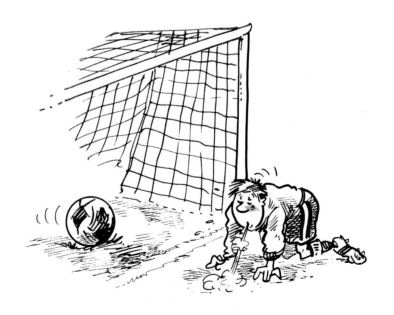

CHESTY COLDS

People talk about colds 'going onto their chest' and being 'chesty'. What does this mean?

Everybody gets colds. When children with asthma get a cold, it makes their asthma worse, and the asthma may continue to be troublesome after the cold has cleared up.

Occasionally children get chest infections caused by viruses or bacteria - acute bronchitis. The symptoms may be very similar to asthma including cough, wheeze and breathlessness, but the difference is this: children do not normally get acute bronchitis more than once or twice a year. If there is repeated cough/wheeze /breathlessness, that is more than twice a year, it's likely to be asthma.

If a child is coughing, what does it matter what medical label you choose? It matters because the treatment for acute bronchitis is antibiotics, which have no effect on asthma. Repeated prescriptions for antibiotics for coughs in children may indicate that the doctor has not really considered asthma.

If asthma is diagnosed, it can be treated effectively.

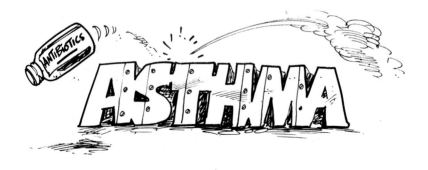

ASTHMA TRIGGERS

All sorts of things can trigger off asthma symptoms, and by observing your child closely you may be able to figure out some of the things that your child is sensitive to. Cough or wheeze or breathlessness linked with a common asthma trigger is a sure sign of asthma.

Whilst the most common asthma trigger is the common cold, other things to watch out for are household pets and horses, pollens and spores (which would tend to cause symptoms over 1 or 2 months) and cold air or sudden changes in air temperature.

We look more closely at asthma triggers in Section 3.

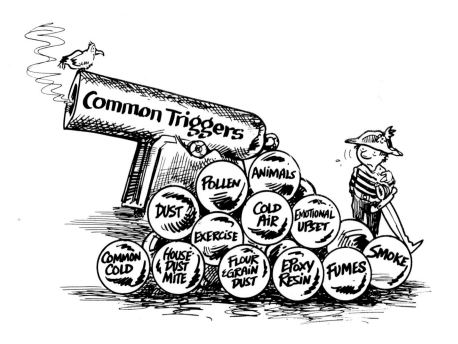

VARIABILITY

Asthma is a condition where the symptoms come and go for no apparent reason. Often the cough will come and go over several weeks or months and may not be obvious on the day the doctor sees your child. (However your story should alert the doctor!) - and if it is asthma the cough will return.

> **What to do if you suspect asthma**
>
> If you suspect your child has asthma, you must go to your family doctor. Only he can provide effective treatment.

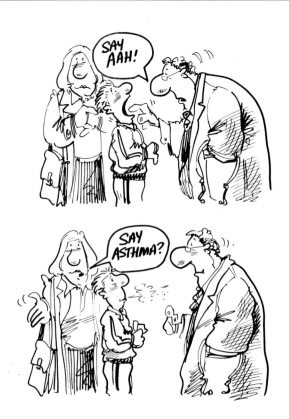

What Causes it?

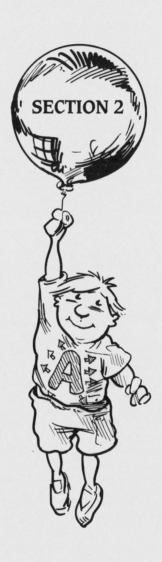

2: WHAT CAUSES IT?

This chapter looks at what goes wrong in the lungs of people with asthma.

On a practical level, you can look after a child with asthma perfectly well without knowing any of this, just as you can drive a car without knowing the first thing about what goes on under the bonnet, so don't feel that you have to master the medical background.

However, many people feel happier if they understand something about the disease that is affecting them or their family, and this chapter provides the background.

THE HEALTHY LUNG

First let's look at the normal lung. When you breathe in, air passes through the nose and mouth into the trachea or wind pipe (trachea = trunk). The trachea divides into main airways or bronchi (bronchus = branch).

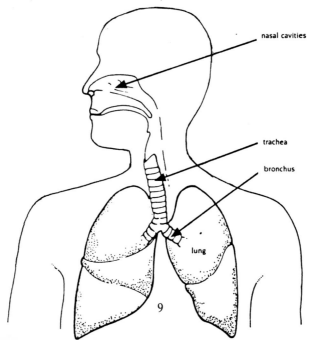

nasal cavities

trachea

bronchus

lung

9

The airways then divide and re-divide into smaller and smaller branches. People often talk of the bronchial tree, although this particular tree is upside down.

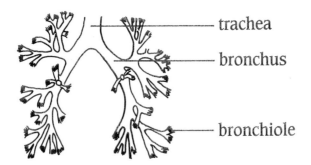

trachea

bronchus

bronchiole

At the end of the smallest airways are air sacs (alveoli) where oxygen from the breathed-in air passes into the bloodstream, and the body's exhaust gas, carbon dioxide, is passed from the bloodstream into the air sacs of the lung to be breathed out.

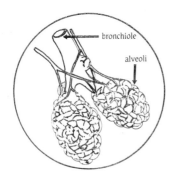

The whole of this respiratory tract, from the nose downwards, is a sort of air conditioning system which takes in every sort of air, hot or cold, clean or dirty, humid or dry, and delivers clean, moist air at body temperature to the alveoli. The airways are lined with soft tissue which produce a sticky substance called mucus: the mucus lines all the airways and serves to trap small dust particles.

Millions of microscopically small hairs (cilia) constantly beat simultaneously at 1,000 times a minute to move mucus towards the top of the trachea where it can be swallowed. Coughing and sneezing also remove excess mucus from the airways.

The outside of the airways is muscle: two sets of muscle fibres which wind down the airways in a double spiral like Greek sandal straps.

BRONCHIAL MUSCLE

When they contract, the airways narrow. These muscles are not under our voluntary control, but in a healthy person they allow the airways to open up slightly during exercise, and close up as a protective mechanism, for example when we go into a smoky room.

So everybody coughs, everybody's airways get narrower sometimes, everybody secretes mucus and this is a normal protective mechanism. In asthma these responses go out of control.

THE LUNG IN ASTHMA

This is what happens during an attack of asthma. The soft tissue lining the airways becomes inflamed and swollen, and this narrows the airways. Too much mucus clogs the airways, and this can completely block some of the smaller ones. The cilia stop beating and sometimes fall off, exposing to the air lung tissue which is normally protected. The airway muscles go into spasm, further narrowing the airways.

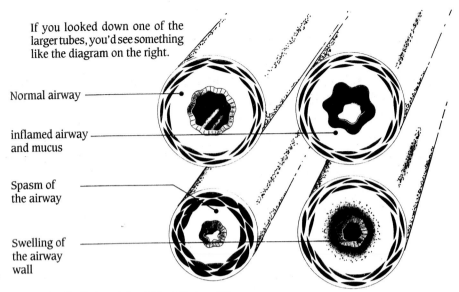

If you looked down one of the larger tubes, you'd see something like the diagram on the right.

Normal airway

inflamed airway and mucus

Spasm of the airway

Swelling of the airway wall

Reproduced by kind permission of Allen & Hanburys Ltd.

So it's not surprising that with all this going on in the lung, people with asthma cough and get short of breath. The wheezing is the sound of air whistling through narrowed airways.

During asthma, it's harder to breathe out than breathe in, because the normal action of breathing in opens up the lungs and compensates a little for the narrowed airways. Many asthmatics describe asthma as 'having your chest blown up with a bike pump' - it's not at all comfortable.

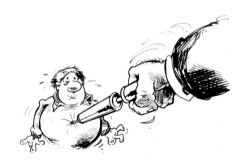

SENSITIVE AIRWAYS

So most of the things that go wrong in asthma - inflammation, mucus production, airway muscle spasm - are normal protective mechanisms gone way out of control.

The difference between asthma sufferers and other people is that they have unusually sensitive airways. Their airways grossly over-react to things that other people's airways can handle such as head colds, pollens or cold air or exercise.

Will he grow out of it?

It's tempting to say yes, and it is true that many children stop having symptoms as they become adults. Asthma is less common in adults than children.

But asthma is a chronic disease, and youngsters who grow out of it by the age of 15, for example, may grow back into it by the age of 35.

The safest prediction is that over the course of a lifetime, there will be times when symptoms are troublesome, and times when symptoms are absent, but the tendency to asthma will always be there.

So you can see, the root cause of asthma is sensitive airways, or 'bronchial hyper-reactivity', not asthma triggers like pollen or horse hair. An asthma attack happens when a person with sensitive airways meets up with an asthma trigger that they're sensitive to:
Airway sensitivity + trigger = asthma.

The hypersensitivity remains, even when the trigger isn't there.

INFLAMED AIRWAYS

In recent years it has become clear that even in between attacks, asthmatics' airways are slightly inflamed and some damage can be seen under the microscope even though there are no symptoms present. It is thought that this low-grade inflammation is linked with the hyper-sensitivity (twitchiness) of asthmatics' airways.

Understanding what goes wrong in asthma helps you understand how the different types of asthma medication work.

Some drugs, when taken regularly, everyday, prevent asthma symptoms before they arise. They reduce the between-attacks inflammation and make the airways less over-sensitive. Examples of these preventive drugs are Intal, Becotide, Beclazone, Filair, Becloforte, Pulmicort and Flixotide - all of which are taken by using one of several varieties of inhaler device.

Another group of drugs relieve asthma symptoms very quickly, and are meant to be taken as soon as symptoms appear. These reliever drugs act mainly on the muscles surrounding the airways, relaxing them and opening up the airway. They have less effect on inflammation.

Common reliever drugs, again inhalers, are Ventolin, Bricanyl, Aerolin, Salamol and Salbulin.

One good reason for treating asthma rather than just putting up with it, is that after a number of years, asthmatics' lungs may become permanently damaged and narrowed, unless the asthma is kept under control.

There's more detail about asthma treatments in Section 4.

All in the Mind?

In the 1960s it was fashionable to see emotional disturbance as the root cause for asthma. Patients were asked about their relationship with their mother and sometimes even referred to psychiatrists. Unfortunately, this idea still persists in the minds of many people, causing unnecessary guilt and confusion, especially for parents. The position as it is currently understood is this:

Emotional upset is one of many factors that can trigger symptoms in an asthmatic person (see Section 3). Usually there are several trigger factors that work at the same time, and emotional upset is only one of them.

Asthmatics have been shown to be no less and no more neurotic than everybody else.

The symptoms of asthma, including disturbed sleep for children and parents, and missing out on normal activities, are in themselves upsetting. Treating the symptoms often removes the emotional problems, but trying to treat the emotional problem does not usually remove the symptoms.

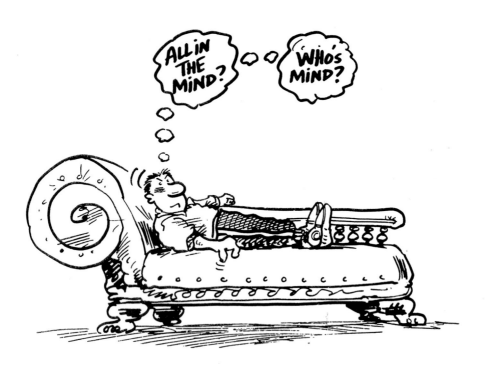

Asthma Triggers

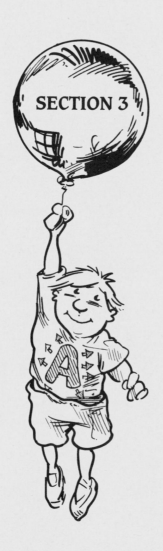

3: ASTHMA TRIGGERS

In section 2 we saw that people with asthma have over-sensitive airways, which respond in an exaggerated and out-of-control way to things that don't bother other people. The things that asthma sufferers over-react to are known as 'asthma triggers', or 'trigger factors'.

There are two ways to deal with trigger factors.

1. Avoid them. This is not always practical or desirable.

2. Pre-empt them by using an anti-asthma medication before exposure to the trigger factor. This means that you have to know what the possible trigger factors are, and what medication to use.

THE COMMON COLD

This is one of the most common triggers. When children with asthma get a cold, it often sets off their asthma symptoms so that even after the cold has gone, the asthma symptoms remain - unless they are treated. Asthma triggered by cold is unfortunately often confused with a chest infection, and antibiotics are prescribed. Antibiotics have no effect on asthma symptoms. Once asthma is diagnosed and the link with the common cold is recognised, the asthma sufferer can increase their preventive medication (see Section 4, Asthma Treatments) as soon as they get their cold, so that asthma is not triggered.

HOUSE DUST MITE

These tiny insects, invisible to the naked eye. They live in carpets, bedding, soft furniture and soft toys, even in the cleanest of houses. They (or rather their droppings) are one of the commonest asthma triggers.

Trying to eradicate house dust mites in your own home (see page 22) may help your child's asthma, but it is unlikely to be the whole answer. Your child will visit other houses, where house dust mites flourish undisturbed, and he will also be sensitive to other trigger factors that you can't avoid. So the message is, that it may be worth trying to attack you house dust mites, but this should be in addition to, not instead of, your standard medical treatment as prescribed by your doctor.

POLLENS AND SPORES

Grass pollens are at their peak in early summer, and this is when hay fever sufferers tend to get their worst symptoms. Asthma sufferers who are sensitive to grass pollen will have asthma in the hay fever season, (unless they are treated) but those who are sensitive to pollens and spores from other plants may have their 'season' at different times.

You can't avoid pollen except by staying inside but you can avoid asking for trouble. For example, if you're sensitive to pollen, it's unwise to roll around in long grass.

If you know when your child's asthma season is, you can make sure he starts a course of preventative treatment before the season starts. In the same way, some of the asthma medications taken before a walk in the country or a picnic will prevent symptoms during and afterwards.

ANIMALS

The hair or feathers and skin debris from household pets are a common asthma trigger: cats, dogs, horses, gerbils, hamsters, rats, guinea pigs, budgies and canaries can all cause problems.

This doesn't necessarily mean that you should dispose of your well-loved pet: there are a lot of other things to take into consideration, including the severity of your child's asthma.

The pet is very unlikely to be the only trigger factor, so by removing the pet you are removing one of many triggers, not the root cause. And the emotional upset that might happen when a child is separated from a pet could also be an asthma trigger.

One answer might be a trial separation, with the pet going to a friend's house or a kennel for a couple of weeks. If, and only if, this was combined with a very thorough spring clean to get rid of all the hair and skin particles that the pet had contributed to the household dust, the trial separation might tell you whether permanent removal would be of any benefit.

As a parent, you already know that very few decisions about your children are easy ones!

However, one can say definitely that if you have an asthmatic child in the family, it is not very sensible to acquire any new pets.

EXERCISE

Almost all asthma sufferers find that the sort of vigorous exercise that makes them breathe hard will bring on asthma symptoms, during and after exercise.

It's not good for your child's health to avoid exercise; asthma symptoms brought on by exercise can be prevented by using the right medication (see Section 4) just before the exercise begins, and by using regular preventative medication.

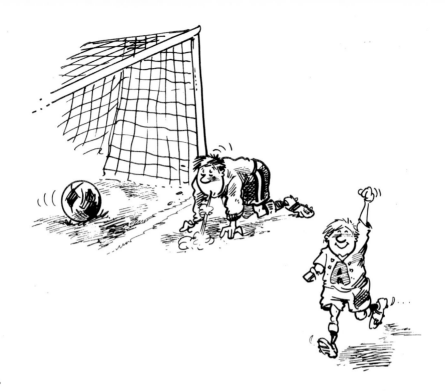

COLD AIR

Going outside on a cold day can set off asthma attacks. Again pre-medication is better than being kept inside. Some people are sensitive to abrupt changes in temperature or humidity.

EMOTIONAL UPSET

The importance of this, can and has been exaggerated (see Section 3). Emotional upset can trigger asthma, but usually it is not the sole factor but one of many.

If you have ever experienced an acute asthma attack, the last thing your want is another one. If a child is upset or under stress, his is much more likely to have an attack even though this is probably the last thing he wants at the time.

For example the child who is having an attack for the first time in two years on the very day his mother starts work outside the home is not having an attack as a method of attention-seeking, but may be worrying about the problems an attack might cause now that his mother has begun to work.

A child who has emotional problems and also has asthma may use their asthma to attempt to manipulate parents and other adults, but would be most unlikely to fake a severe attack.

LESS COMMON ASTHMA TRIGGERS

There are a number of substances that are known to trigger asthma and they are officially recognised for the purposes of compensation for industrial injury. It is possible that your child may be exposed to these at home or in school.

★ Epoxy resins (in adhesives, paints and plastic)

★ Colophony fumes (from soldering)

★ Grain or flour dust

★ Wood dust

FOOD ALLERGY

Food allergy is not a common asthma trigger. However, it does occur occasionally. Sometimes the food in question is obvious, and the allergic reaction includes a skin rash: some types of nuts, fruit or shellfish can have this effect. Here the remedy is easy - avoid that food. If you suspect from careful observation that some more common foodstuff may be linked with your child's asthma, you may need expert advice from a specialist, and your first stop is your family doctor.

DUST AND SMOKE

Dust and smoke make lots of people cough and tend to have a worse effect on people with asthma. Cigarette smoke is a very strong trigger for asthma and parents who smoke will certainly make their children's asthma worse.

DEALING WITH TRIGGERS

Many asthmatics know what triggers their attacks, and the vast majority can identify several triggers that apply to them. In practical terms, this means that eliminating triggers is not a very effective way of treating asthma; if the horse hair doesn't get you, the house dust mite will, and if the house dust mite doesn't get you, the head-cold will, etc., etc.

It's more logical, and more effective, to tackle the over-sensitivity which makes asthmatic airways respond to trigger factors, and modern preventive medications (see Section 4) can do just that.

However, very rigorous dust control in the home has helped some individual asthma sufferers, and you may feel you would like to give it a try. It won't do any harm but it's hard work and costs money. This is what you do:

-   Replace divan beds with slatted wooden beds.

-   If possible buy new mattresses.

-   Cover the mattresses in plastic sheeting.

-   Replace any feather pillows and eiderdowns and woollen blankets with synthetic ones.

-   Change the bedlinen weekly.

- Remove carpets, soft toys and animals from the bedroom.

- Place soft toys in the freezer for at least six hours a week, and then vacuum clean them.

- Change to a vacuum cleaner that returns very low amounts of dust to the room (see Which, May 1992).

- Change to light, washable curtains or blinds.

This will reduce, but not eliminate, the house dust mite, but will not affect any other possible triggers. All this may help your child's asthma.

Desensitization treatment did enjoy a vogue but is rarely used in this country now. Once you know what the asthma sufferer is sensitive to the idea is to inject larger and large quantities of that substance (extract of cat fur, horse hair, grass pollen, etc.); this has the effect of reducing the patient's sensitivity to that substance.

On the whole, this treatment was less effective than standard anti-asthma drugs, and could be very dangerous. It is possible to develop a very serious allergic shock reactions to this treatment, even several hours after the event, and there have been deaths. And you can't even attempt to desensitize people to the common cold, cold air or emotional upsets.

Asthma and Allergy

There is a link between asthma, hay fever and eczema. Asthma sufferers, and their relatives, tend to suffer from hay fever and eczema, and all these conditions can be triggered off by allergic reactions to substances such as grass pollen, house dust mite and pet hair. Sometimes doctors use skin tests to discover who is allergic to what substances. Tiny amounts of pollen or house dust mite are injected under the skin, and if you are allergic to a substance, a weal will form at the site of the injection. 90% of asthmatics test positively for at least one of the four main allergens - grass pollen, house dust mite, pet hair or skin, and the common mould aspergillus fumigatus.

People who test positively on skin tests, or who have a family history of allergic diseases are known as atopic individuals. Atopy is the potential to develop allergy as distinct from allergy itself.

This is very interesting, but not very helpful to people with asthma. Many, but not all, asthmatics are atopic. Even when the allergies are known, they are not usually the only thing that trigger asthma - most children's asthma is also triggered by exercise, cold air and the common cold. 25% of the whole population are atopic and only a minority of these people have hay fever or asthma.

Asthma Treatments

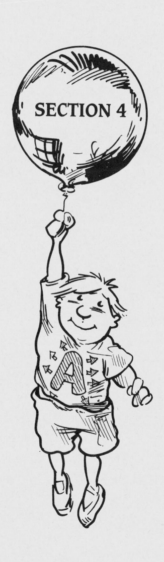

4: ASTHMA TREATMENTS

There is no permanent cure for asthma, but with modern treatments the vast majority of asthmatics can remain free of symptoms and lead completely normal lives. But many people with asthma, even those who have been correctly diagnosed, are not getting the most effective treatment and continue to suffer symptoms - cough, wheeze, shortness of breath, tightness in the chest, disturbed sleep and restricted physical activity.

Parents who are well-informed about asthma can ensure that their child receives the best available treatment.

PREVENTION

These days it can be quite confusing to know what treatment has been prescribed because each drug can have at least two names. The generic name (basic drug name) and a brand name (the manufacturer's name) (see Appendix 1 - Section 4).

Some types of asthma medication prevent asthma symptoms occurring, but do not relieve symptoms when they occur. The most common are inhaled steroids and sodium cromoglycate. The table over the page shows you examples of preventer therapies and the inhalers through which the treatment is delivered.

Preventer inhalers come in several different colours, including white/grey, white/red, brown, maroon and orange but are never blue.

DELIVERY OF PREVENTIVE MEDICINES VIA DIFFERENT INHALER DEVICES

Examples of most commonly prescribed therapies

DEVICE	INHALED STEROID	SODIUM CROMOGLYCATE
Metered Dose Inhaler	Becotide Beclazone Becloforte Filair Pulmicort Flixotide	Intal Cromogen
Syncroner		Intal
Autohaler	Aerobec Aerobec forte	
Easi-Breathe	Beclazone	
Spinhaler		Intal
Rotahaler	Beclotide	
Turbohaler	Pulmicort	
Diskhaler	Becotide Becloforte Flixotide	
Accuhaler	Flixotide	
Volumatic Spacer	Becotide Becloforte Flixotide	
Nebuhaler Spacer	Pulmicort	
Fisonair Spacer		Intal

See Appendices 2-13 for more information on devices.

Preventive treatments only work if they are taken regularly and can take a little time before they are fully effective. Sometimes it may take a few days, others several weeks.

The point about preventive medication is that after a few days your child will feel well, and may forget to take their medication or consider that he has better things to do. This is how controllable asthma begins to get out of control again.

The word steroid often strikes fear into the heart of patients, especially parents of asthmatic children. This is probably because steroid tablets are linked in people's minds with severe and unpleasant side-effects.

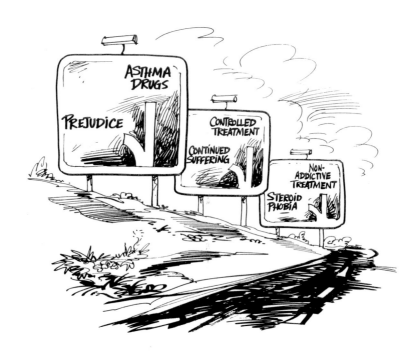

Let's get things in proportion. Inhaled steroids are prescribed in micrograms, steroid tablets in milligrams. A microgram is a thousandth of a milligram, so you can see the doses of inhaled steroids are tiny compared with the tablets.

The reason that such extremely low doses are effective is that the inhaler delivers the drug particles straight to the lung, just where they are needed.

Inhaled steroids have been very widely used since 1976, and the only common side-effects are hoarseness, and sometimes a fungal infection in the throat. Both problems are uncommon in children and can generally be prevented in one of three ways by swilling out the mouth, and/or cleaning the teeth after taking the treatment and/or using the inhaler before food.

So, if your doctor suggests inhaled steroids for your child's asthma, be reassured that these are highly effective, well-tried and tested medicines, and at least give them a try, for a month or so, before deciding (after discussion with your doctor) that this is not what you want for your child.

Sodium cromoglycate is not a steroid, belonging to a completely different chemical family. There are virtually no side-effects, except that the dry powder form of the drug occasionally makes some people cough when they inhale it. Sodium cromoglycate is sometimes the first line of preventative therapy, and can be very effective. The only way of finding out whether it is effective in you child is to use it regularly for a few weeks and see what happens.

RELIEF

Some asthma medicines give almost immediate relief of mild asthma symptoms. They are usually blue inhalers - blue = relief. The most common names are Ventolin, and Bricanyl.

DELIVERY OF RELIEVER MEDICINES VIA DIFFERENT INHALER DEVICES

Examples of most commonly prescribed therapies

DEVICE	RELIEVER
Metered Dose Inhaler	Ventolin Bricanyl Salbulin Airomir Salamol
Autohaler	Aerolin
Easi-Breathe	Salamol
Rotahaler	Ventolin
Turbohaler	Bricanyl
Volumatic Spacer	Ventolin
Nebuhaler Spacer	Bricanyl

See Appendices 2-13 for more information on devices.

Exercise

All these relief drugs, and Intal, will prevent asthma brought on by exercise if taken before the exercise starts.

These inhalers are very quick and effective in relieving asthma symptoms and have made a big difference to thousands of people's lives. The most common side-effect is slight tremor of the hands. This is not dangerous and the main problem with reliever inhalers is that people might place too much reliance on them and use them in the wrong way. There are two situations to watch out for:

1. In a really bad attack (see Section 7) there's a temptation to keep using the trusty blue inhaler even though it doesn't seem to be doing much good. This can waste valuable time and cause people to delay calling out the doctor or going to hospital when they really need to.

2. If you need to use a relief medicine (blue inhaler) every day, or almost every day, it really is more logical and probably more effective, to use instead a preventive medicine like inhaled steroids or sodium cromoglycate. The blue inhalers are best reserved for occasional use, when asthma symptoms 'break through' the preventive cover, or for children who only get symptoms now and then.

Although these reliever inhalers act quickly, their effects only last for about 4 hours, so to keep symptoms at bay you may have to use them several times a day. Even then the last dose at night will have worn off by the early hours, which is the worst time for many asthma sufferers. Regular doses of preventive medicines, on the other hand, should stop symptoms occuring.

Atrovent (ipratropium bromide) is also an inhaled drug which relieves asthma symptoms, but it acts in a different way to the others mentioned here and its effect is not so rapid. It is sometimes used for very small children.

Serevent (salmeterol) is a long acting reliever and should only be used in conjunction with inhaled steroids to give additional relief. Salmeterol can be given via the metered dose inhaler, the Diskhaler or the Accuhaler.

In summary, you can see that it's important to get clear whether the asthma medication prescribed for your child is for relief or prevention, because these are different groups of drugs, with different actions, used in different ways.

BRONCHODILATOR - TABLETS AND SYRUP

A number of the same medicines that are used in reliever inhalers are available in the form of syrup or tablets - Ventolin, Bricanyl, Volmax. Some doctors prescribe syrups for very young children who can't manage inhalers, although wherever possible an inhaler device should be tried (more about inhalers can be found later in this section).

The tablets are usually of a special kind which release the drug slowly, so that its effect lasts far longer than the 4 hours you get from a blue inhaler. This is particularly useful in dealing with night-time symptoms, where you want the effect of the night-time dose to last until morning.

Both tablets and syrup act more slowly than inhalers, beginning to work after hours rather than minutes. Although these are the same drugs that are used in reliever inhalers, the syrups and tablets are intended to be taken regularly, to prevent symptoms. They act too slowly to give quick relief. The disadvantage of all the tablet and syrup asthma drugs is that to achieve the same effect in the lungs as an inhaled drug, you need to use many times the dose. The recommended dose of salbutamol inhaler is 0.1 mg (100 micrograms), whereas salbutamol tablets are 4 mg. This means that side-effects are more common with tablets than with inhaled therapy. This is why most doctors prefer the inhaled route whenever possible.

THEOPHYLLINE TABLETS

There are lots of different brands: the most common are Theo-Dur, Uniphyllin Continus, Slo-Phyllin and Nuelin.

They all contain the drug theophylline in a slow release formulation, so that 2 daily doses give 24-hour cover.

Doctors may prescribe theophylline tablets as an alternative to inhalers, or as an addition to them, or when night-time symptoms are especially troublesome.

Theophylline although an effective asthma drug, is used less often than relief inhalers and prevention inhalers as it is quite a difficult drug to use. Perhaps it should be reserved for the more severe asthmatic child who is being followed up at a hospital clinic.

What's difficult is achieving the right dose that is high enough to be effective, but not so high as to cause side-effects. Unless the doctor actually takes regular blood samples to measure the concentrations of theophylline in the blood (and in practice this is rarely done), he has to start with a low dose and proceed by trial and error.

The side-effects of theophylline may include nausea and other tummy upsets, rapid pulse and palpitations, headache and sleeplessness. Some studies in school children in the USA (where theophylline is used more widely than in Britain) indicate that it may be associated with learning and behaviour problems, such as restlessness, irritability and poor concentration.

EMERGENCY DRUGS

If somebody is admitted to the hospital with a severe asthma attack, they will be given very high doses of inhaled relief treatment such as salbutamol, and a large dose of steroid tablets: yes, it's that dreaded word again.

Steroid tablets are the most effective way to quickly get rid of the inflammation and mucus (phlegm) that clogs up the airways in a severe asthma attack.

And a short, sharp course of steroid tablets is the most effective way of preventing a bout of asthma from developing into a really serious, even fatal attack. People who are subject to severe asthma attacks (see Section 7) are sometimes given an emergency supply of steroid tablets (prednisolone or prednesol) by their doctor and told to start taking them as soon as symptoms start getting worse. A typical dose would be 20-30 mg a day.

Now if you took 30 mg of steroids a day for several months you would certainly experience some unpleasant side-effects, but in asthma we are only talking about a week or two at the most. High doses of steroids for a short period of time are not dangerous, and have a dramatic effect on severe asthma. It is also interesting to note that they will work better taken all at once in the morning after breakfast. Although of course, they can be taken at any time in the 24 hours if necessary.

So, if your doctor prescribes a short course of prednisolone or

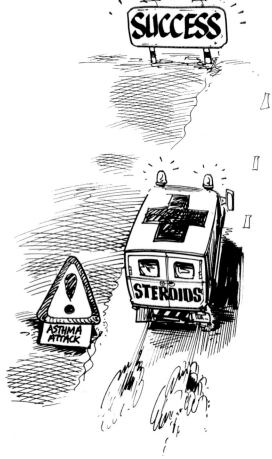

prednesol tablets for your child, there is no need to be worried about long-term side-effects. The steroids will quickly restore lungs back into a more normal condition, and then you can stop the steroid tablets and use other treatments to keep the lungs working well.

Regular steroid tablets, at a lower dose, are reserved for those rare people with very severe asthma which cannot be controlled by other medication.

FALLACIES AND PHOBIAS

Many parents with children with asthma are understandably worried about their child taking any form of medication on a regular basis for a number of years.

It's certainly a good principle to try to control asthma symptoms with the 'minimum force', but some parents, for the best of motives, carry this principle too far, subjecting their child to asthma symptoms which could have been avoided.

"I don't want to weaken his resistance", is what some parents say. They think that asthma drugs are like alcohol: the more you have, the more you need to get the same effect. This is not true of asthma drugs. They are not addictive, and you don't need to keep increasing the dose to get the same effect. Not using asthma drugs will not increase your child's 'natural resistance'. In fact if anything the reverse is true - if asthma is left untreated, it can eventually lead to permanent narrowing of the airways.

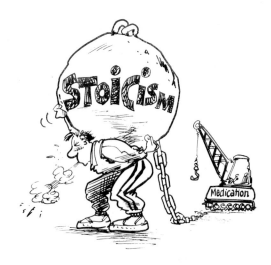

'Steroid phobia' in parents sometimes gets in the way of effective asthma treatment for their children. The word 'steroid' is so loaded that even otherwise reasonable parents refuse to accept reasoned argument and well-established facts. In a similar way some parents withhold relief asthma treatment if they are needed for relief of symptoms. There is no benefit from withholding treatment when symptoms appear. With the best of intentions, they are putting their own prejudices above their child's health.

INHALERS

Inhaling asthma drugs rather than swallowing them has two big advantages.

1. The dose is at least 10 times smaller, so there are very few side-effects.

2. Relief drugs act much more quickly.

The snag is that it's a lot easier to swallow a tablet or a spoonful of syrup than to use an inhaler device correctly. To use an inhaler the doctor or nurse has to teach, and the patient has to learn, a certain technique. Even when this technique has been learned, it's easy to fall into bad habits. When asthma medicines seems not to be working, very often it's because the patient's inhaler technique is faulty in some way. This means that the drug ends up in the back of the throat, or the stomach, rather than in the lung.

For these reasons, a great deal of effort and ingenuity has gone into designing inhaler devices that are simple to use. Most children fare far better using a simple device rather than the standard metered dose inhaler. We show you here the most common devices, with some instructions on how to use them. If your child uses an inhaler, you should check from time to time that he's using it properly, by comparing what he does with the instructions. Your doctor or practice nurse should also be checking inhaler technique at regular intervals. See Appendices 2 - 13 starting on page 42.

Stigma

Some children may feel that using an inhaler device, which is a less discreet procedure than taking a tablet, is not cool. Worries about street cred may be enough to deter them from using their inhaler when they should, especially if they have to do it in front of their peers. Parents should be sensitive to children feeling stigmatised and try and arrange for privacy if there is a need for it.

INHALERS AND PRE-SCHOOL CHILDREN

With a standard inhaler, you have to breathe out, then inhale the drug deeply, then hold your breath. This is too complicated for very young children, and babies can't understand the instructions (believe it or not there are many adults including doctors, who never master the technique).

In practice this means that babies and young children often get tablets or syrup rather than inhaled therapy, but there are now several ways of providing inhaled therapy even for very young children.

With a spacer device like the Volumatic (Appendix 4, page 44), Nebuhaler (Appendix 5, page 45), an adult can spray the correct dose of drug into the spacer device, and the child can inhale it just by breathing normally through the mouthpiece - no need for any special breathing technique. Of course not all children can be persuaded to breathe through the mouthpiece.

To cater for this, there are now special face-masks available which fit onto the mouthpiece of the spacer device. This means that, if your child will accept having the face mask on for a few minutes, the inhaled drug can be delivered. There is a new spacer device for very small babies called the Babyhaler which may be purchased. We recommend that before you buy one you should talk to your doctor or asthma nurse.

Using a spacer may seem all a bit of a fuss, but if it enables you to control your child's asthma using 10 times less medication, isn't it worth it?

NEBULISERS

Some children with asthma may use nebulisers to deliver asthma drugs. Nebulisers are machines (usually electric) which, through a compressor, transform a drug solution into a fine aerosol mist which can be breathed in by normal breathing via face mask or mouth piece. Nebulisers are another way of enabling very young children to benefit from inhaled therapy.

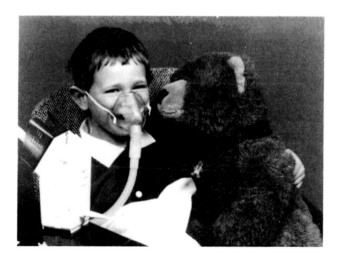

The advantage of nebulisers is that they do not require any special technique and they can deliver much larger doses than ordinary inhaler devices. They are not however very easy to carry around.

Nebulisers are useful for a very small number of asthma sufferers, but they are not the be all and end all. Indeed, their very effectiveness can be a danger as people can rely on them too heavily, failing to call their doctor or call the hospital when they need to. Just like any other person with asthma, those who use nebulisers need to know how to use their medication, when to increase it or decrease it, and when to call for help.

COMPLEMENTARY MEDICINE

There are many asthma treatments of offer outside the NHS, which we group together under the heading 'complementary medicine'.

Of course there isn't a great divide between mainstream medicine and complementary medicine. For example, there's a group of potential anti-asthma drugs under research at the moment which derive from the ginkgo tree, used in Chinese herbal medicine for centuries.

The main difference between 'complementary' medicine and mainstream medicine is that for a drug to be available for prescription, it has to go through a very rigorous series of trials in animals and humans, to show that it is both effective and reasonably safe. Something from the health shop has not been through this procedure. This is not to say it won't work for you: it just happens that this product has not had sufficient investment behind it to put it through long and very expensive trials. If you try complementary medicines it is important not to stop conventional treatment without consulting your doctor.

What follows is not an exhaustive list, but a mention of some of the non-prescription products that are marketed, in some cases quite aggressively, to people with asthma. Whatever the claims are, none of these products has been through a proper clinical trial with the results published in a scientific journal, so, although they may give benefit to some individuals, it is impossible to give any general recommendation.

Ionisers: There is no evidence to prove they are of benefit but there is some evidence to show that these actually increase night-time cough.

Face-masks: Are meant to filter out dust particles.

Special Vacuum Cleaners such as Medivac: These are supposed to have better filters than ordinary vacuums and allow less dust to recirculate back into the air. A Which? report of May 1992 looked at a whole range looked at a whole range of vacuum cleaners, including these special ones. It might be wise to try an ordinary vacuum cleaner with low dust emission, to see if this has any effect on symptoms, before deciding on a more expensive specialist model.

Actomite is an insecticide spray which claims to reduce the house dust mite population. There is no scientific evidence for any general benefit to asthma sufferers.

Some makers of air conditioning and filtration systems and even insecticidal paint are making claims about asthma, but there's no proof that they do any good.

	BRAND NAMES	BASIC NAME
Preventers	Intal Cromogen	Sodium Cromoglycate
	Becotide Becloforte Aerobec Beclazone Filair	Beclomethalone Diproprionate
	Pulmicort	Budesonide
	Flixotide	Fluticasone Propionate
Relievers	Ventolin Salamol Salbulin Aerolin Airomir	Salbutamol

HOW TO USE A
METERED DOSE INHALER

1. Remove the cap and shake the inhaler.

2. Breathe out gently.

3. Put the mouthpiece in the mouth and at the start of inspiration, which should be slow and deep, press the canister down and continue to inhale deeply.

4. Hold the breath for 10 seconds, or as long as possible.

5. Wait several seconds before taking another inhalation.

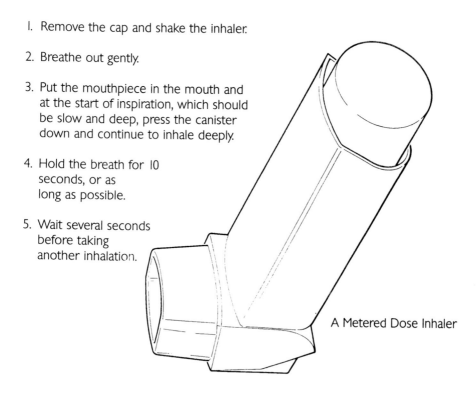

A Metered Dose Inhaler

HOW TO USE THE
AUTOHALER DEVICE

1. Remove protective mouthpiece and shake the inhaler.

2. Hold the inhaler upright and push the grey lever right up.

3. Breathe out gently. Keep the inhaler upright and put the mouthpiece in the mouth and close lips round it. (The air holes must not be blocked by the hand).

4. Breathe in steadily through the mouth. DON'T stop breathing when the inhaler 'clicks' and continue taking a really deep breath.

5. Hold the breath for about 10 seconds.

6. Wait several seconds before taking another inhalation.

7. N.B. The lever must be pushed up ('on') before each dose, and pushed down again ('off') afterwards, otherwise it will not operate.

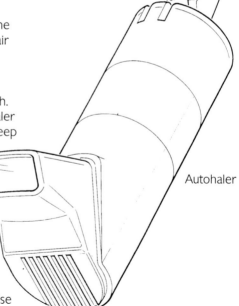

Autohaler

HOW TO USE A SPACER DEVICE
e.g. VOLUMATIC
Method for patients who can use the device without help

1. Remove the cap, shake the inhaler and insert into the device.

2. Place the mouthpiece in the mouth.

3. Press the canister once to release a dose of the drug.

4. Take a deep, slow breath in.

5. Hold the breath for about 10 seconds, then breathe out through the mouthpiece.

6. Breathe in again but do not press the canister.

7. Remove the device from the mouth.

8. Wait about 30 seconds before a second dose is taken, and repeat sections 1-7.

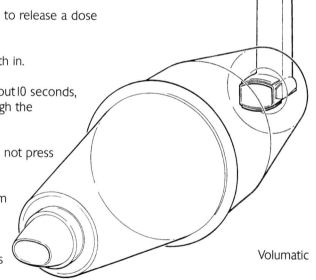

Volumatic

HOW TO USE A SPACER DEVICE
e.g. NEBUHALER
Method particularly useful for young children

I. Remove the cap, shake the inhaler and insert into the device.

2. Place the mouthpiece in the child's mouth, (if using the Nebuhaler be careful the child's lips are <u>behind</u> the ring).

3. Seal the child's lips round the mouthpiece by gently placing the fingers of one hand round the lips.

4. Encourage the child to breathe in and out slowly and gently. (This will make a 'clicking' sound as the valve opens and closes).

5. Once the breathing pattern is well established, depress the canister with the free hand and leave the device in the same position as the child continues to breathe (tidal breathing) several more times.

6. Remove the device from the child's mouth.

7. For a second dose wait 30 seconds and repeat sections 1-6.

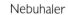

Nebuhaler

HOW TO USE THE FISONAIR

1. Line up the notches on the two halves of the Fisonair and push together firmly.

2. Remove the cap from the inhaler, shake and insert into the device.

3. Breathe out gently (but not fully).

4. Place the mouthpiece in the mouth.

5. Holding the device level, press the canister once to release a dose of the drug.

6. Breathe in slowly and deeply.

7. Remove the device from the mouth.

8. Hold the breath for ten seconds, or as long as is comfortable.

9. If a second dose is required wait about one minute before repeating stages 2-8.

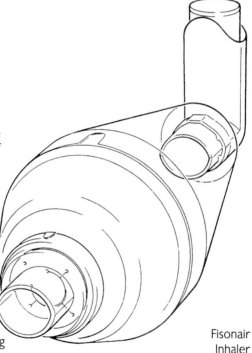

Fisonair
Inhaler

HOW TO USE THE ROTAHALER

1. Hold Rotahaler vertically and put capsule (clear end first) into 'square' hole. Make sure top of Rotacap is level with top of hole. (If there is a Rotacap already in the device this will be pushed into shell).

2. Hold Rotahaler horizontally, twist barrel sharply forwards and backwards. This splits capsule into two.

3. Breathe out gently. Keep Rotahaler level and put mouthpiece between lips and teeth and breathe in the powder quickly and deeply.

4. Remove Rotahaler from the mouth and hold breath for about 10 seconds.

5. If any powder is left repeat steps 3 and 4

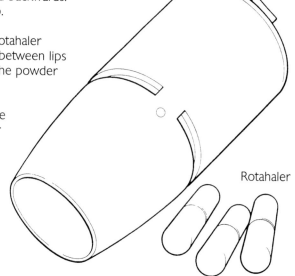

Rotahaler

HOW TO USE THE SPINHALER

1. Hold Spinhaler upright with the mouthpiece downwards, and unscrew the body.

2. Put <u>coloured</u> end of spincap <u>into cup</u> of propeller, making sure it spins freely.

3. Screw the two parts together and hold horizontal. Move grey sleeve up and down once or twice, this will pierce capsule.

4. Breathe out gently, tilt the head back, put Spinhaler into the mouth so the lips touch the flange and breathe in quickly and deeply.

5. Remove Spinhaler from the mouth and hold breath for about 10 seconds, and then breathe out slowly.

6. If any powder is left in the spincap, repeat steps 4 and 5 until it is empty.

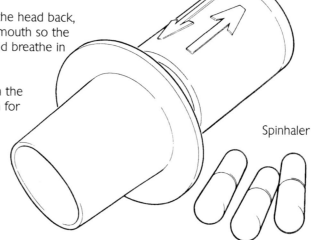

Spinhaler

HOW TO USE THE DISKHALER

TO LOAD

1. Remove mouthpiece cover. Then remove white tray by pulling it out gently and then squeezing white ridges either side until it slides out.

2. Put foil disk - numbers uppermost - on wheel and slide tray back.

3. Holding corners of the tray, slide tray in and out to rotate disk until number 8 shows in window.

TO USE

1. Keeping the Diskhaler level, lift rear of lid up as far as it will go, to pierce top and bottom of blister. Close the lid.

2. Holding the Diskhaler level, breathe out gently, put mouthpiece in the mouth and breathe in as deeply as possible. (Do not cover the small air holes on either side of the mouthpiece).

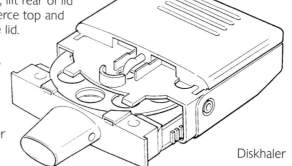

Diskhaler

3. Remove Diskhaler from the mouth and hold breath for about 10 seconds. Slide tray in and out ready for next dose.

HOW TO USE THE TURBOHALER

1. Unscrew and lift off white cover.
   Hold Turbohaler upright and twist the grip forwards
   and backwards as far as it will go.
   You should hear a click.

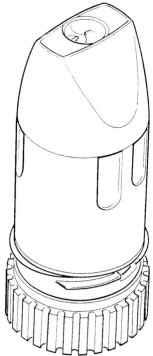

Turbohaler

2. Breathe out gently, put the
   mouthpiece between the lips
   and breathe in as deeply as
   possible. Even when a full
   dose is taken there may be
   no taste.

3. Remove the Turbohaler from
   the mouth and hold breath
   for about 10 seconds.
   Replace the white cover.

HOW TO USE THE ACCUHALER

TO USE

1. Hold the outer casing of the Accuhaler in one hand whilst pushing the thumbgrip away until a click is heard.

2. Hold Accuhaler with mouthpiece towards you, slide lever away until it clicks. This makes the dose available for inhalation and moves the dose counter on.

3. Holding Accuhaler level, breathe out gently away from the device, put mouthpiece in mouth and suck in steadily and deeply.

4. Remove Accuhaler from mouth and hold breath for about 10 seconds.

5. To close, slide thumbgrip back towards you as far as it will go until it clicks.

6. For a second dose repeat sections 1 - 5.

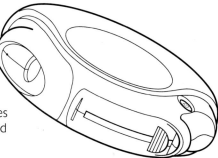

Accuhaler

HOW TO USE THE
SYNCRONER INHALER

1. Remove the green mouthpiece.

2. Lift the canister holder until it clicks into position.

3. Shake the inhaler well (at least 5 times).

4. Holding the inhaler well away from the mouth, breathe out gently but not fully.

5. Put the mouthpiece in the mouth and at the start of inspiration, which should be slow and deep, press the canister down and continue to inhale deeply.
   (If no spray is seen to escape from the syncroner then the dose has been taken correctly.)

6. Hold the breath for about 10 seconds.

7. Wait one minute, then repeat steps 3-6 before taking another inhalation.

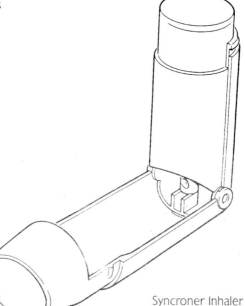

Syncroner Inhaler

HOW TO USE THE EASI-BREATHE

TO USE

1. Shake the inhaler.

2. Hold the inhaler upright. Open the cap.

3. Breathe out gently. Keep the inhaler upright, put the mouthpiece in the mouth and close lips and teeth around it (the airholes on the top must not be blocked by the hand).

4. Breathe in steadily through the mouthpiece. DON'T stop breathing when the inhaler "puffs" and continue taking a really deep breath.

5. Hold the breath for about 10 seconds.

6. After use, hold the inhaler upright and immediately close the cap.

7. For a second dose, wait a few seconds before repeating sections 1 - 6.

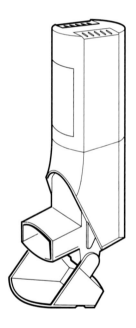

Easi-Breathe

Fine Tuning

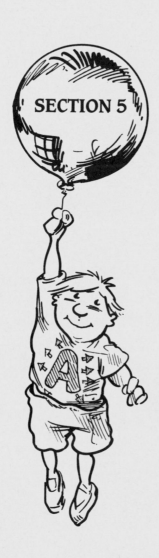

5: FINE TUNING

Asthma is a variable disease: symptoms come and go, sometimes in time with the seasons or the weather, sometimes for no apparent reason. Managing asthma is a bit like trimming the sails on a yacht - you have to make frequent adjustments and always keep alert to changing circumstances. The idea is to decrease dosages if you can, but increase dosages, when you have to, so as to keep asthma symptoms well under control, and avoid any serious attacks.

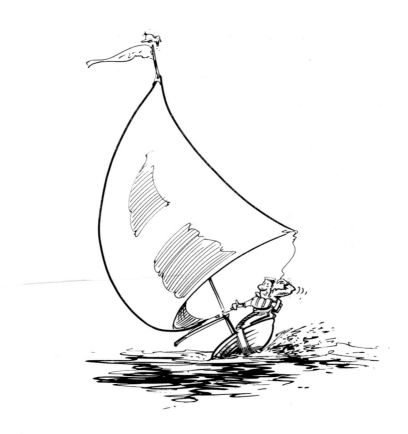

MANAGEMENT PLANS

Ideally, you will have worked out with your GP or asthma nurse an asthma management plan for your child. This will tell you, in writing:

- what drugs to take when, at what dosage.
- what signs and symptoms of worsening asthma to look out for.
- when to increase or decrease the dose of regular medication.
- when to call the doctor.

Even if you haven't got such a plan, there's nothing to stop you asking your doctor for this information and writing it down yourself.

WORSENING ASTHMA

The common signs of worsening asthma are:
- ★ increased symptoms - cough/wheeze/breathlessness.
- ★ increased symptoms during or after exercise.
- ★ reliever medicines seem to work less well, or are needed more often.
- ★ disturbed sleep.

If you have a management plan, it should cover these situations and you should know what action to take.

If you don't have a management plan, or if you aren't clear about what to do, arrange to see your doctor or asthma nurse. Don't wait for things to get even worse. If your doctor thinks you're making a fuss about nothing, that's his problem. It's better to see your doctor in the surgery about worsening asthma than to call him out in the middle of the night for a really severe attack.

MEASURING LUNG FUNCTION

Some children with asthma are encouraged to measure their lung function, twice daily or more, and adjust their asthma therapy accordingly. The idea is to predict a worsening of actual symptoms before it happens, and nip it in the bud by increasing the dose of preventive asthma medication.

HOW TO USE
THE PEAK FLOW METER

1. Stand up if possible.

2. Check cursor is on zero.
    (L/Min position)

3. Take a deep breath in and place Peak Flow Meter in the mouth (hold horizontally), and close lips.

4. Blow suddenly and hard.

5. Note number indicated by cursor.

6. Return cursor to zero.

7. Repeat twice and obtain three readings.

8. Write down the best of the three readings.

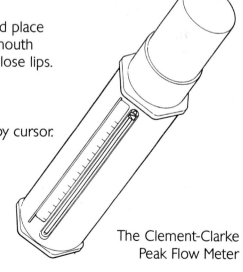

The Clement-Clarke
Peak Flow Meter

Lung function is measured by using a peak flow meter. What is measured is Peak Expiratory Flow (PEF) - in other words how hard you can blow out - in litres per minute. A healthy adult can usually manage 500 - 600 L/min, obviously for children this is much less and will depend on how tall they are.

Some people keep a peak flow record card which charts the progress of their asthma and the response to treatment.

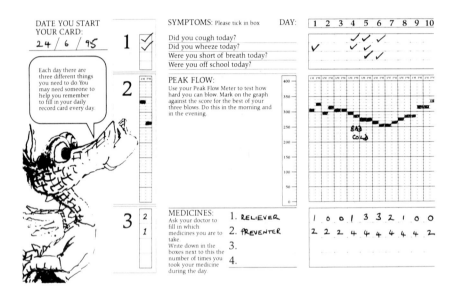

For an asthmatic, recording peak flow is just as important as measuring blood sugar is for a diabetic and they should be given every help and encouragement.

But measuring and recording peak flow is not an end in itself - it's pointless unless you know what action to take at what levels of peak flow. It is also of no value if your child does not use the meter properly. Most children under the age of six will not produce accurate readings.

Children and parents should know:

- How to measure peak flow correctly (see page 56).

- What to do at given levels of peak flow.

These instructions are different for every child. Your doctor or clinic may give you peak flow values at which to increase preventive medication, start oral steroids or call for emergency help. If ever you are not sure what to do, contact your asthma nurse or doctor immediately - better safe than sorry.

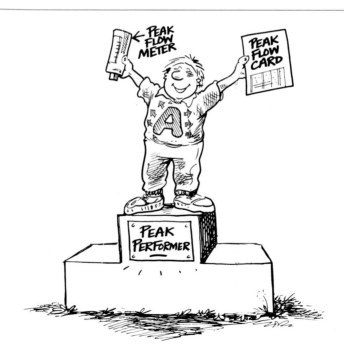

NOTE: Is is more important for a young child to know how to use an inhaler device than a peak flow meter. Some children understandably get confused about blowing and sucking and in this case sucking is more important.

Living with Asthma

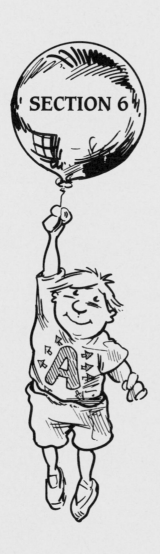

6: LIVING WITH ASTHMA

In theory, with modern treatments, there is no reason why the vast majority of children with asthma should not be completely free of symptoms virtually all the time, and lead completely normal lives.

In practice, quite a few things get in the way of providing ideal asthma treatment, and this chapter deals with some of them.

SCHOOL

If your child has asthma, he may need to use his inhaler at school - for example relief medication or sodium cromoglycate before playtime or a games lesson, or sodium cromoglycate at lunchtime as part of regular preventive treatment. (Inhaled steroids need only be taken morning and evening and so shouldn't need to be taken during school time.)

Some schools have strict policies about medicines, and your child may have to give his inhaler in to the school office, then go and ask for it when he needs it. From the school's point of view, this guards against the whole playground having a puff of the inhaler, but from your child's point of view, it's an obstacle to proper treatment. Especially if he feels well, all the bother of going to the office and finding his inhaler may be a less attractive proposition than whatever's going on in the playground.

If your child is subject to asthma attacks in the daytime, it is the school who will have to deal with the situation. It's important that the correct medicine is available, and that the school knows how to recognize a serious attack, what to do, and when to call you and/or the doctor.

It is a good idea to talk to your child's class teacher about his asthma, and ask

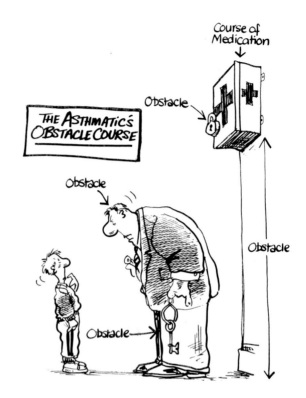

- Does my child have free and easy access to their asthma medication?

- Do you and other teachers know what to do in the event of an asthma attack?

The National Asthma Training Centre (address at the back of this book) has produced a special book for schools called 'Asthma Who Cares? - at School'.

SCHOOL ASTHMA CARDS

Asthma treatment can be complex, and teachers can't be expected to remember details of treatment for each child - there may be several in each class. To aid communication between school, home and surgery, the National Asthma Campaign (see back of the book for address) have produced a School Asthma Card which doctors or nurses can fill in to provide an authoritative record of what treatment is needed when, for each child.

SCHOOL TRIPS

School trips and residential courses present a special challenge to children with asthma and those who care for them. The excitement and change in routine may cause children to forget to take medicines, and there may be greater exposure to some trigger factors, for example grass pollen at a school camp. The best way to encourage children to cope with this challenge is for the parents of the children with asthma to provide the teacher in charge with a management plan for the treatment of their asthma. This plan would include not just details of medicines, but what medicines should be used 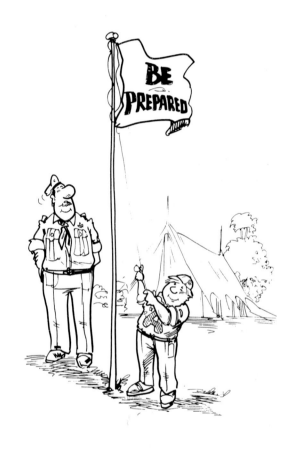 when, and when to seek help. If you can't provide a management plan, you should see your family doctor or asthma nurse. (See Section 5, Fine Tuning.)

SPORTS AND EXERCISE

Asthma is not a reason for not doing any sport of activity, and asthmatics can count among their number many world class sportsmen and women. As with many things, it's not what you do, but the way you do it.

The problem to be overcome is exercise-induced asthma: breathlessness, perhaps combined with cough and wheeze, during hard exercise and after it. The abrupt change from warm to cold air can make things worse.

Regular preventive medication will help prevent these symptoms and may well abolish them altogether, but exercise-induced asthma might sometimes break through this protective cover. In this case, blue relief inhalers, or Intal, before the exercise starts and before going out into cold air will do the trick. It sounds simple, but needs a bit of organisation. In particular teachers and other adults at school need to understand what your child needs to do, and when, and ideally should remind children with asthma to take their blue inhaler before exercise.

People with asthma seem to tolerate swimming better than some other activities, perhaps because the air is moist and warm, but with proper treatment, people with asthma can tackle anything. There's no reason to force an unwilling child to swim rather than play football just because he has asthma.

SMOKING

For an asthmatic to smoke is particularly self-destructive.

★ In the short term it makes asthma symptoms worse. Smoke is a trigger factor.

★ In the long term many smokers develop chronic bronchitis: chronic bronchitis is mainly a disease of smokers. Like asthma, this causes cough and breathlessness, but the breathlessness is there all the time, the drugs are much less effective than in asthma, and the damage done to the lungs is irreversible. To have asthma and chronic bronchitis is often very disabling.

Inhaling someone else's cigarette smoke makes asthma worse. There is increasing evidence that exposure to cigarette smoke before birth and during the first year of life increases a childs' tendency to develop asthma and other chest diseases. The residue of smoke in a room and even on clothing can have a detrimental effect. These are excellent reasons for anybody who has contact with a child to give up smoking. They are not only damaging their own health but also that of the child and are setting a bad example.

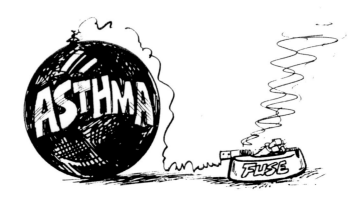

Smoking is a difficult habit to break but is always well worth the effort. If you have tried unsuccessfully to stop your family doctor and his team may be able to offer you help.

YOU AND YOUR DOCTOR

By now you will have understood that we are not pretending that every GP always knows everything and always makes the right decision.

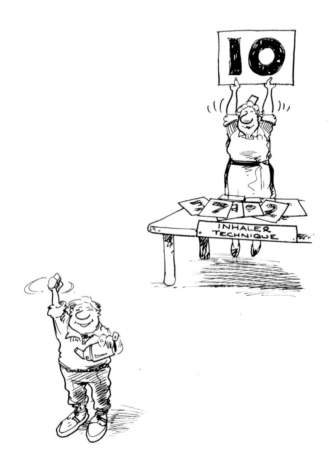

The plain fact is that some GPs, and some GP practices, are better at managing asthma than others. To be good at managing asthma you have to be interested in it. It takes a lot of time (perhaps 30 minutes to do an initial assessment, for example) and there are lots of asthma sufferers in every practice. Asthma is not high on every GPs list of priorities, so not every GP will devote the necessary time to it himself, or will take the trouble to organise routine asthma management in co-operation with a specially-trained nurse.

You will reach your own conclusions about how well your own family doctor and his team are managing your child's asthma. If you are not satisfied, you are perfectly entitled to change to another practice, without giving any reason. All you have to do is go to the new practice and ask them to take you on.

If a practice runs special asthma clinics, or has a specially trained practice nurse who routinely sees asthma patients, it's a sure sign that the practice has thought carefully about asthma and is interested in it. This doesn't mean that a practice without an asthma clinic or a trained nurse isn't keen on asthma management. Try and talk to other patients in the practice who have asthma.

The Asthma Attack - What to Do

SECTION 7

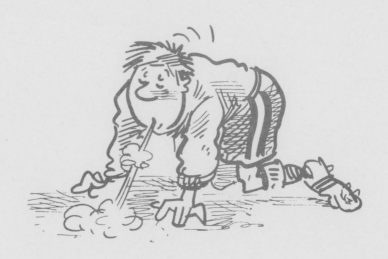

7: THE ASTHMA ATTACK - WHAT TO DO

The whole point of effective asthma management is to avoid asthma attacks, but they may still happen. This is a checklist of what to do. If your child is subject to severe attacks, you should talk to your family doctor and plan what to do, together, in advance.

Ideally your management plan for asthma should cover acute attacks and tell you what to do. (See Section 5, Fine Tuning.) If you do not have a management plan, follow the advice below.

If a child with asthma becomes breathless and wheezy or coughs continually:

1. Keep calm. It's treatable.

2. Let him sit down: don't make him lie down.

3. Give him his blue inhaler.

4. Wait 5-10 minutes.

5. If the symptoms disappear, the child can go back to what he was doing.

6. If the symptoms have improved, but not completely disappeared, give another dose of inhaler and keep a close eye on the child.

7. If the normal medication has had no effect, see severe asthma attack below.

WHAT IS A SEVERE ASTHMA ATTACK?

Any of these signs means severe:

1. Normal medication does not work at all.

2. The child is breathless enough to have difficulty in talking normally.

3.   Distressed breathing.

4.   Pallor or change in colour.

5.   Extreme lethargy/drowsiness.

(Your doctor or nurse will advise you, if it is appropriate, to estimate the severity by checking the child's peak flow rate.)

HOW TO DEAL WITH A SEVERE ATTACK
Either follow your management plan or:

1.   Call the family doctor.

2.   Ask him to come immediately.

3.   If he is reluctant, take the child to the nearest hospital casualty department straight away and get someone to warn them you are coming. Alternatively call an ambulance.

4.   If the child has an emergency supply of oral steroids (prednisolone, prednesol) give the stated dose to the child **now**. These are vital, but will not have an effect for at least an hour.

5.   Keep trying with the usual reliever inhaler, and don't worry about possible overdosing.

ISN'T THIS OVERDRAMATIC?

2,000 people die from asthma each year, and the vast majority of these deaths are avoidable.

An important factor in many deaths is that patients, relatives and carers underestimate the seriousness of the situation and delay seeking treatment.

EMERGENCY TREATMENT VIA VOLUMATIC

I. Put 2 parts of spacer (Volumatic) together.

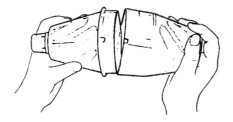

2. Remove cap of inhaler

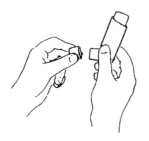

3. Shake inhaler.

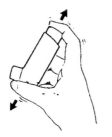

4. Insert inhaler into flat end of device.

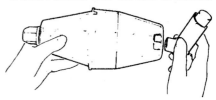

5. Push down inhaler canister once to release dose of reliever (Ventolin).

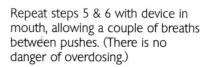

6. Place mouthpiece in mouth Slowly breathe in and out of the spacer device.

Repeat steps 5 & 6 with device in mouth, allowing a couple of breaths between pushes. (There is no danger of overdosing.)

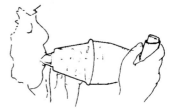

7. Remove device from mouth.

WHILE HELP IS BEING SOUGHT REPEAT STAGES 5-7 UP TO 15-20 TIMES IN AN EMERGENCY

EMERGENCY TREATMENT
VIA NEBUHALER

NB. The Nebuhaler is provided with an of additional white plastic inhaler for the aerosol. If this has not already been removed, then remove it before following the procedure below.

I. If not already assembled, put 2 parts of spacer (Nebuhaler) together.

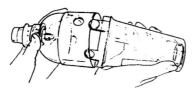

2. Remove cap of inhaler.

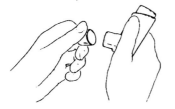

3. Shake inhaler.

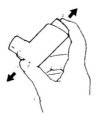

4. Insert inhaler into flat end device.

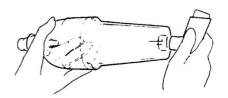

5. Push down canister once to release dose of reliever (Bricanyl).

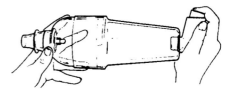

6. Breathe slowly in and out of the spacer device.

Repeat stages 5 & 6 with device in mouth allowing a couple of breaths between pushes. (There is no danger of overdosing.)

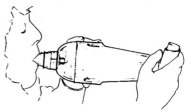

7. Remove device from mouth.

WHILE HELP IS BEING SOUGHT REPEAT STAGES 5-7 UP TO 15-20 TIMES IN AN EMERGENCY

"What a Wheeze"
&
"Huffin Puffin"
Educational Material
for Schools and
the Home

'Huffin Puffin's Asthma Activity Book'
- designed to make learning
about asthma fun -

*For further information and order forms
please write to:-*

National Asthma Training Centre
Winton House, Church Street,
Stratford-upon-Avon, CV37 6HB.

Telephone: (01789) 296974